SUPERHERO SCIENCE

SUPER HEALI

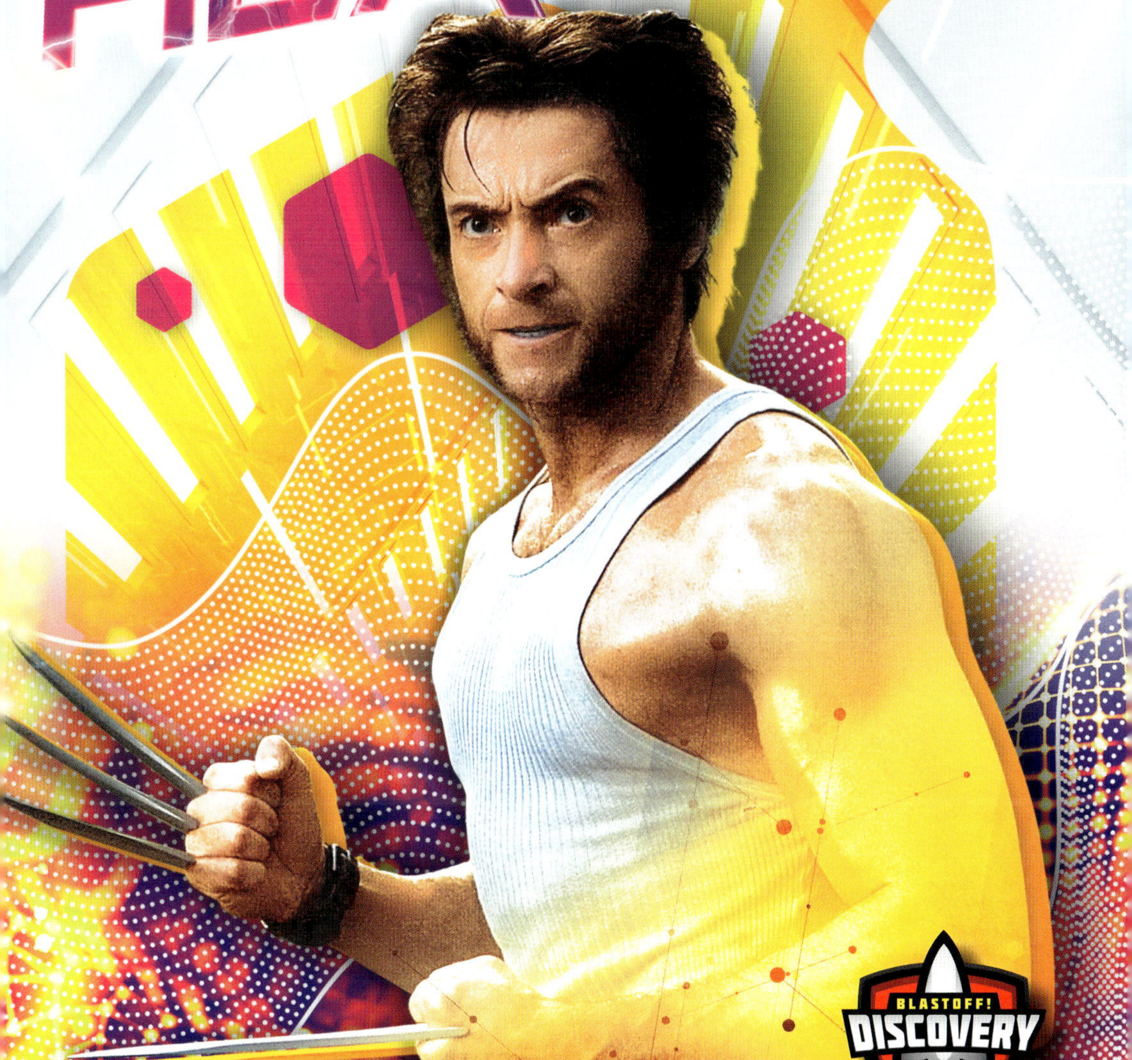

BLASTOFF! DISCOVERY

BY BLAKE HOENA

BELLWETHER MEDIA • MINNEAPOLIS, MN

This edition first published in 2022 by Bellwether Media, Inc.

Library of Congress Cataloging-in-Publication Data

LC record for Super Healing available at: https://lccn.loc.gov/2021049542

Editor: Elizabeth Neuenfeldt Designer: Andrea Schneider

Printed in the United States of America, North Mankato, MN.

TABLE OF CONTENTS

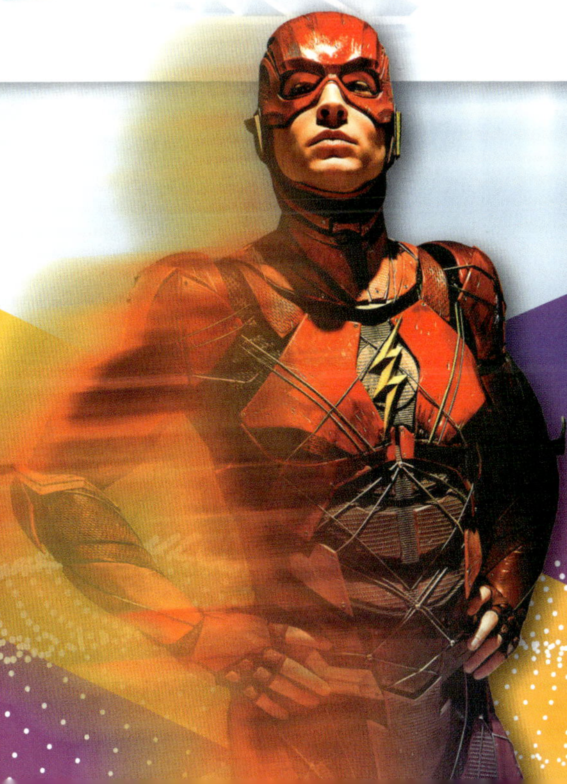

A MAGICAL HEALER

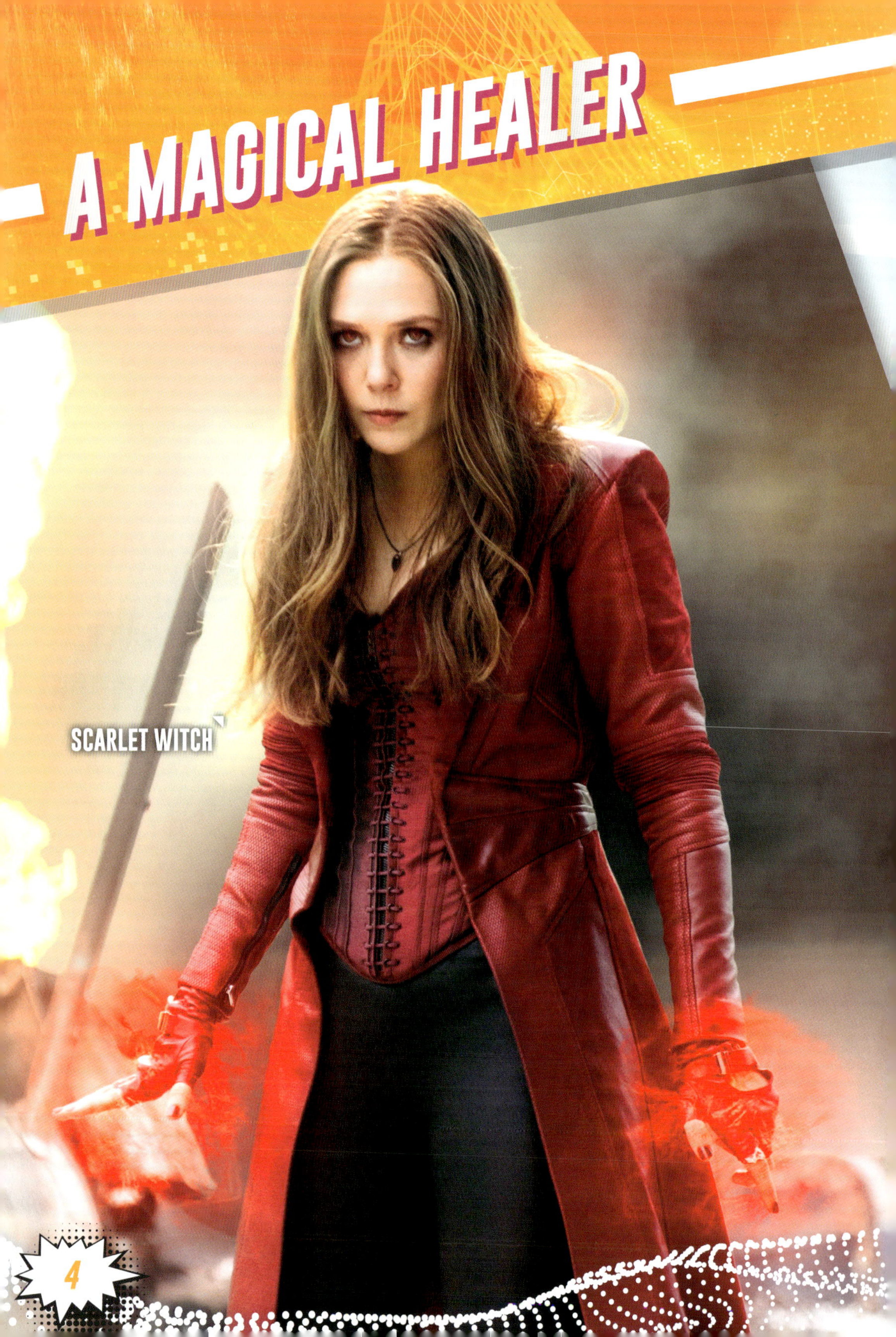

Wanda Maximoff walks down the city streets. The people around her do not know that she has a secret identity. She is a superhero! Wanda is the Scarlet Witch, a powerful **sorcerer**.

Suddenly, there is a huge explosion behind her. People are thrown to the ground. Bricks and concrete rain down all around. Buildings are set on fire. The Scarlet Witch knows danger is near. Her hands begin to glow red as she prepares to use her magic.

SUPER SIBLINGS

The Scarlet Witch has a brother. His name is Pietro Maximoff. He is better known as Quicksilver, a superfast superhero!

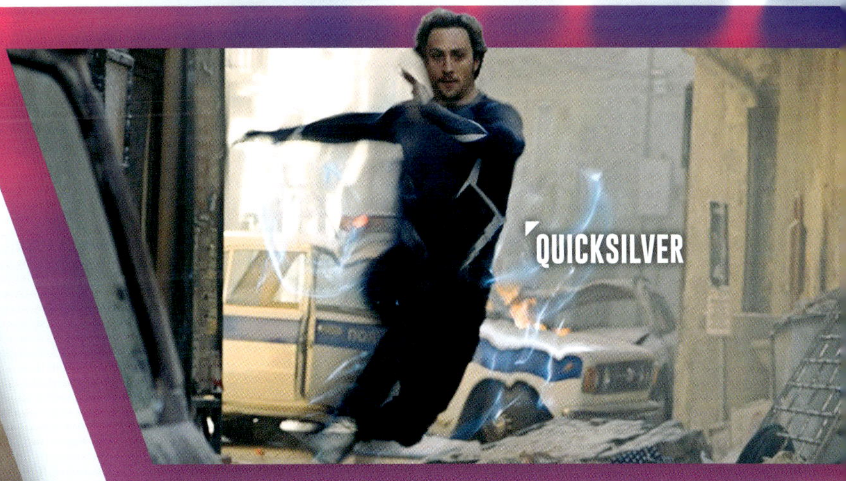

Hawkeye comes running down the street. He is a superhero and an expert archer. He tells the Scarlet Witch that Ultron is attacking the city. The heroes go to stop the evil robot! Hawkeye fires exploding arrows at Ultron. The Scarlet Witch uses her magic to attack the robot.

Then, Ultron strikes Hawkeye with a crushing blow. The hero flies through the air and falls to the ground. The Scarlet Witch rushes over to Hawkeye. He is seriously hurt. The Scarlet Witch uses her magic to heal the fallen superhero. Her healing powers save his life!

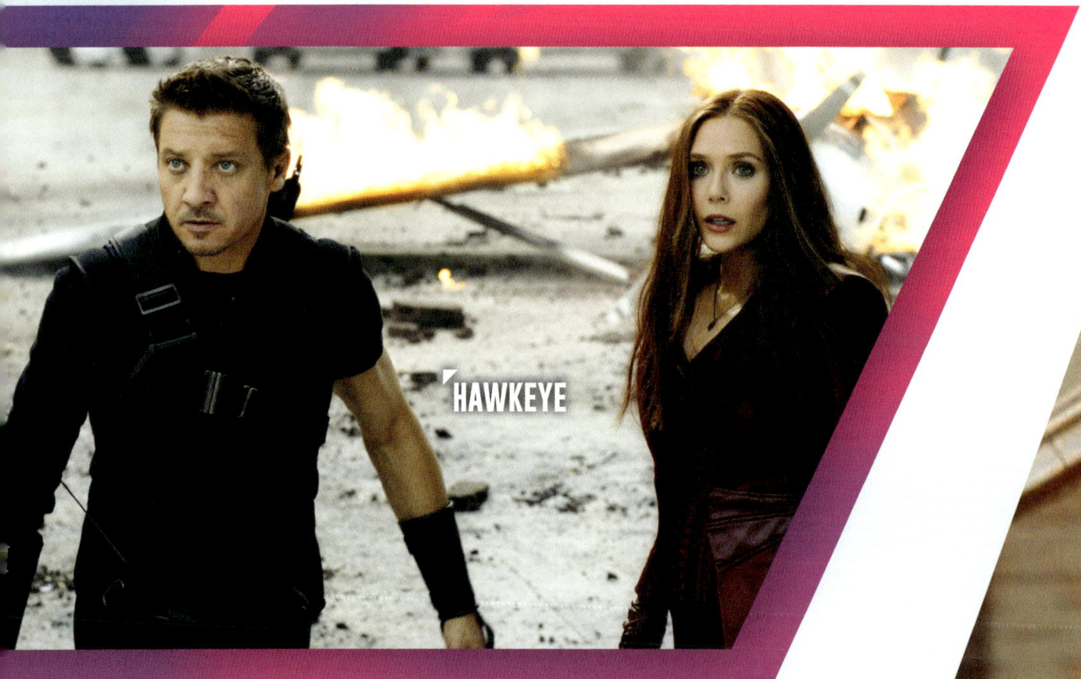
HAWKEYE

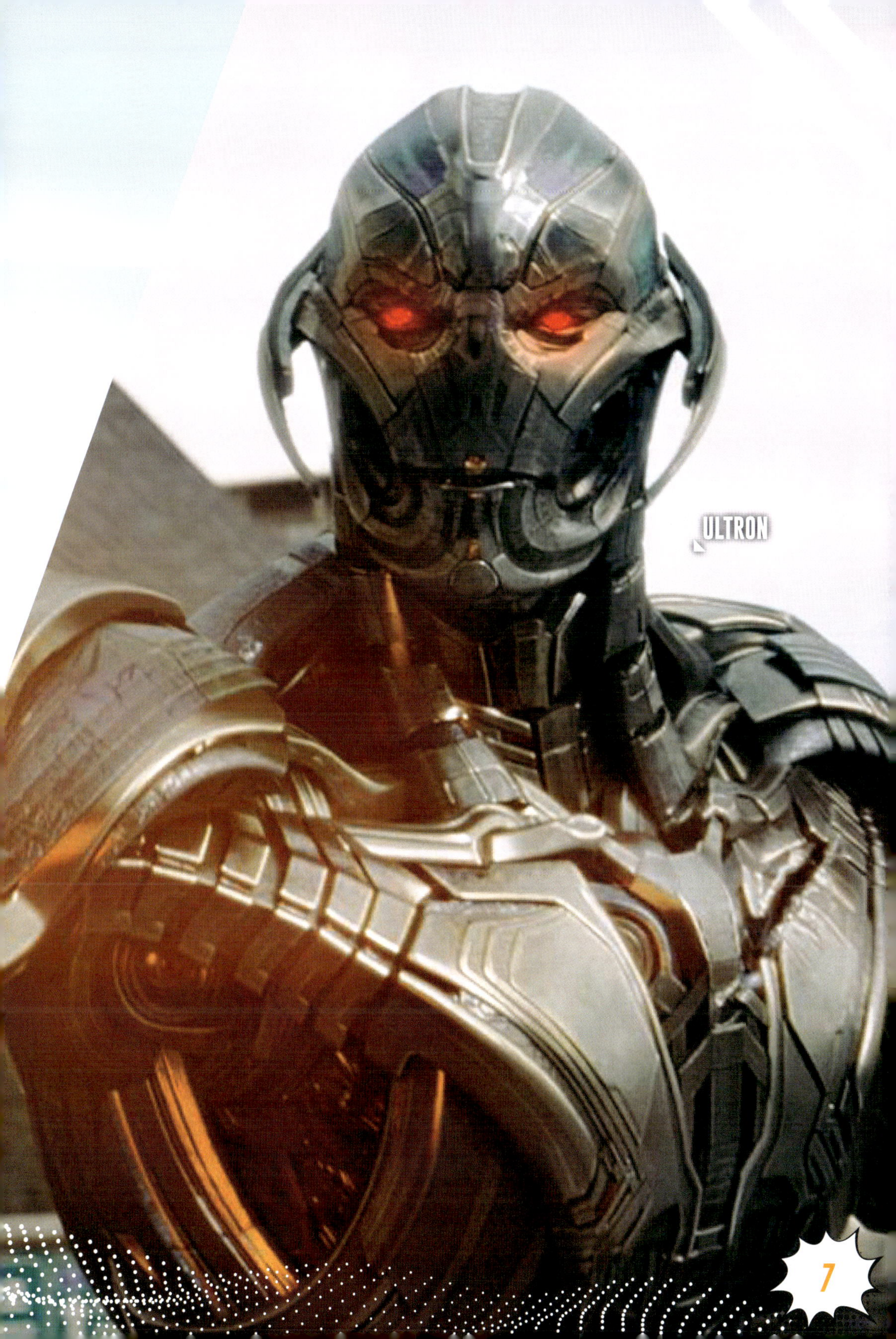
ULTRON

THE SUPERPOWER OF HEALING

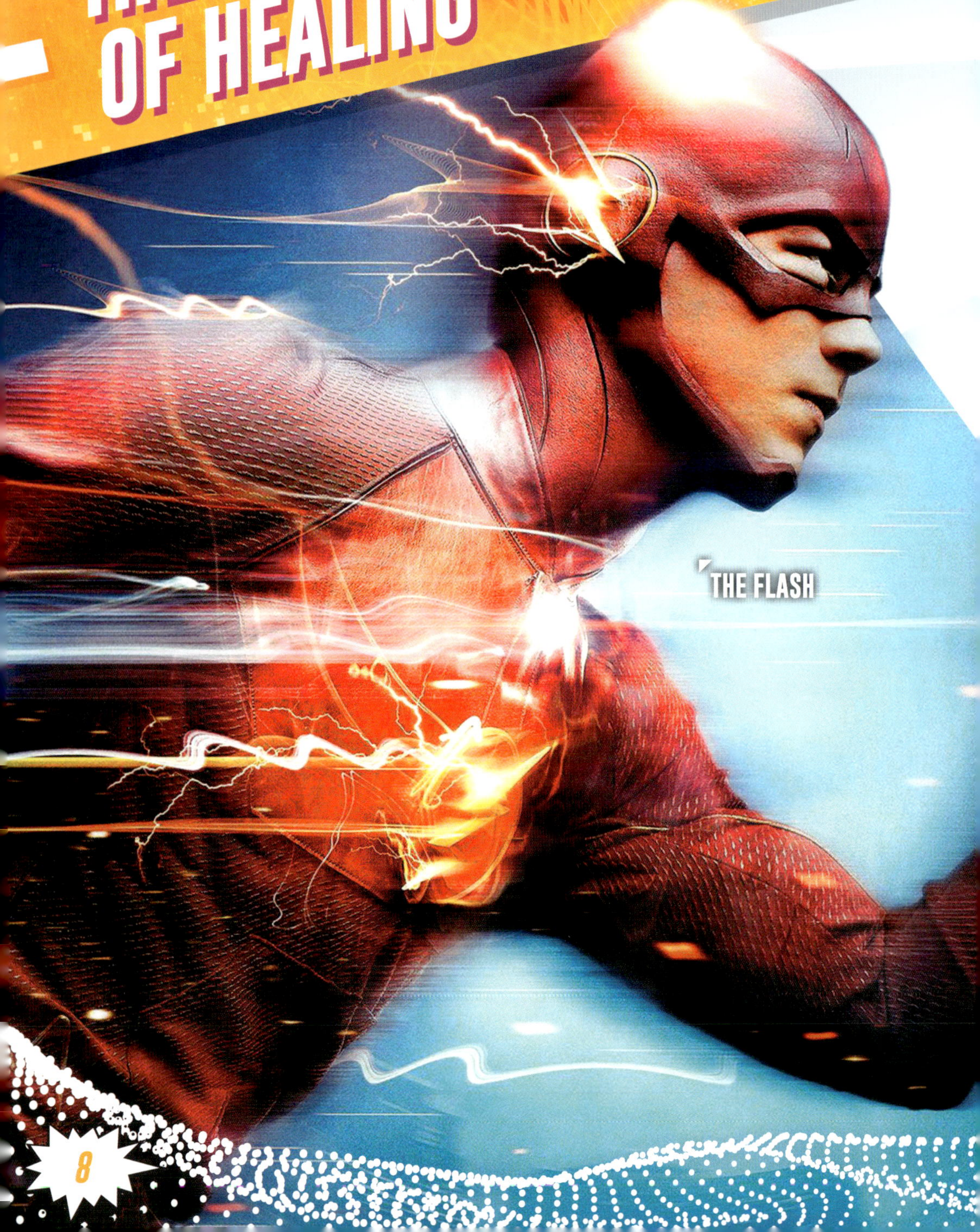

THE FLASH

Super healing is the **ability** to cure diseases and heal wounds. Some superheroes, like the Scarlet Witch, can heal other people. Other heroes, like the Flash, can quickly heal their own bodies.

The Flash sped into DC comic books in the 1940s. Along with running superfast, he quickly heals from injuries. The Flash can recover from cuts and bruises almost instantly. He can heal a broken bone in hours!

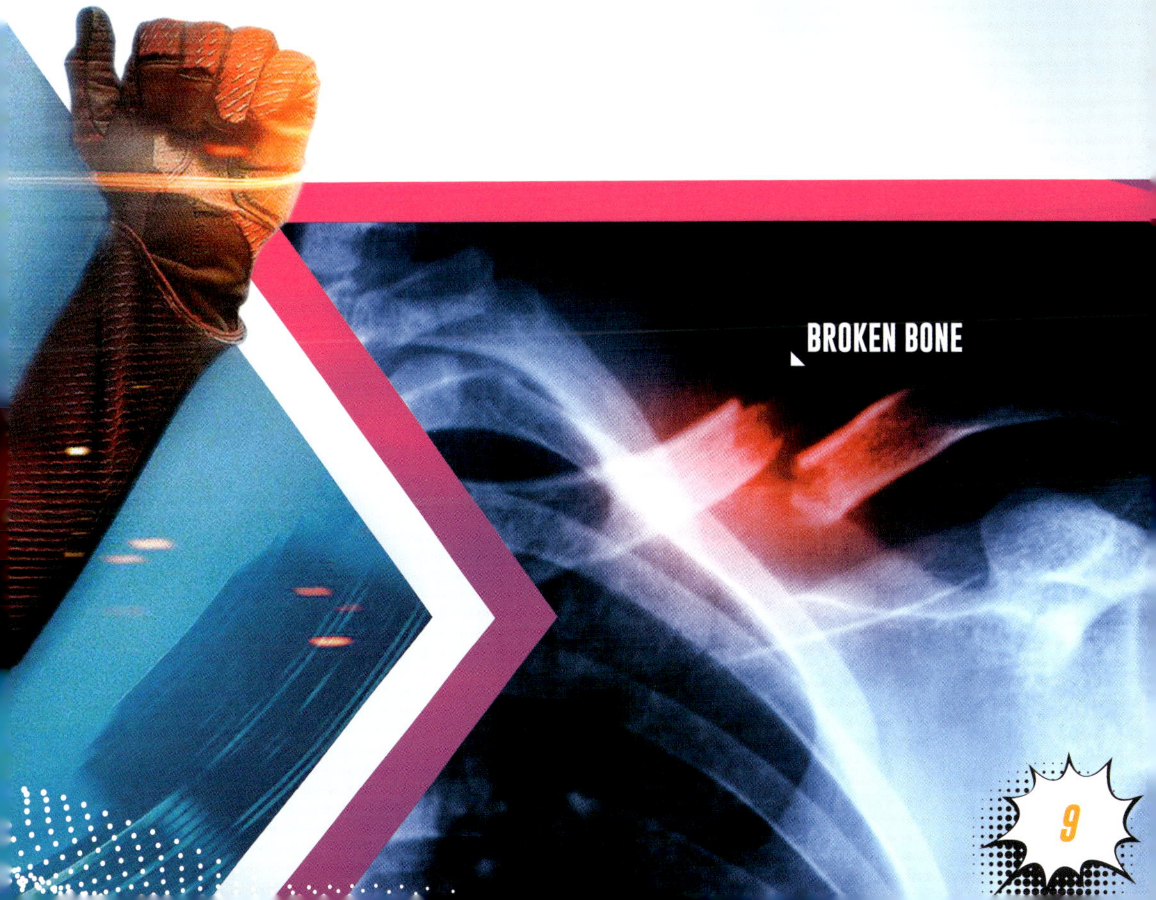

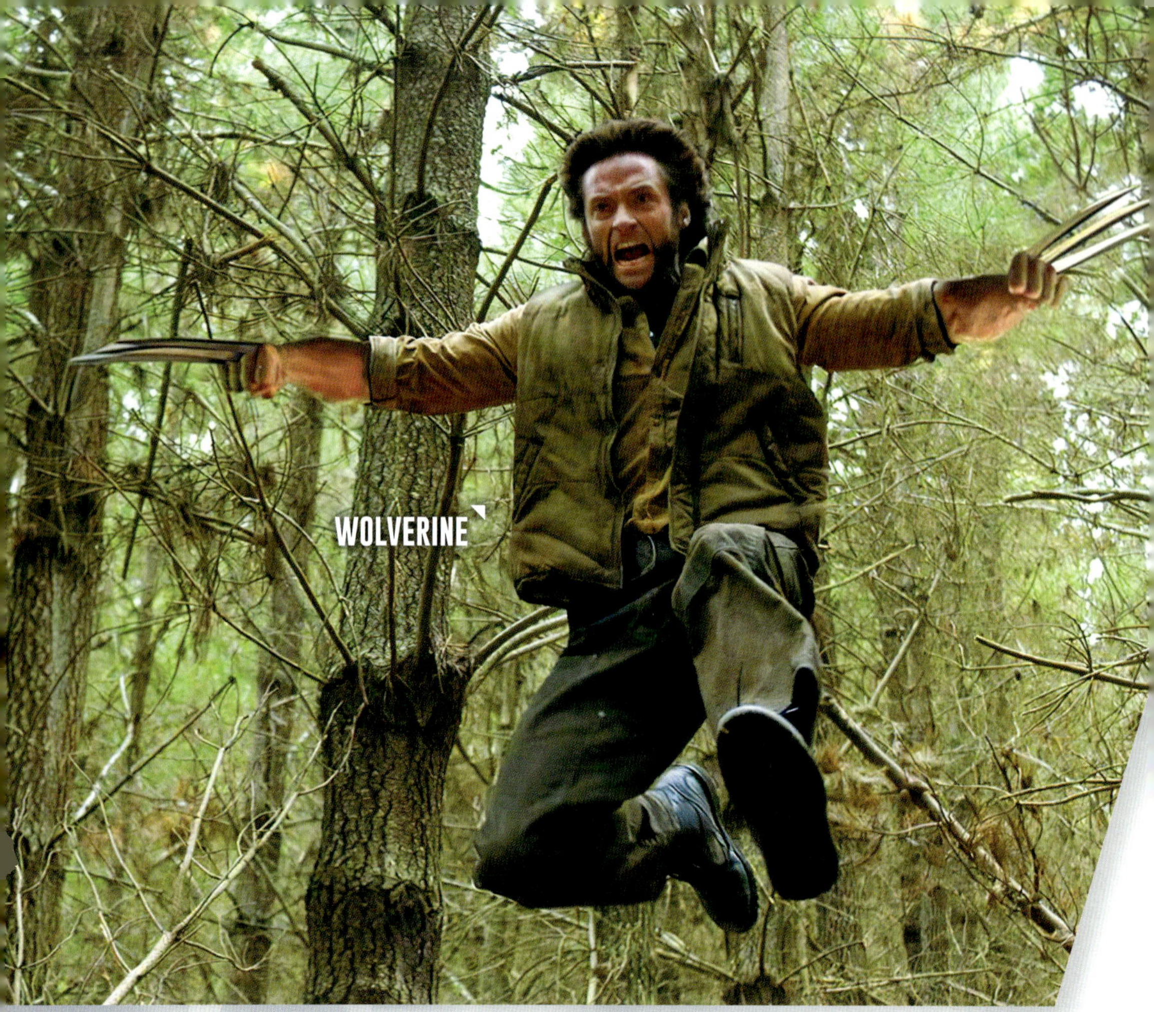

Over time, more healing heroes were made. In the 1970s, Marvel introduced comic book readers to Wolverine. He is best known for the claws that extend from his fists. But he can also quickly regrow body parts. He can heal from almost any injury!

In the 1980s, Jennifer Walters first stomped across Marvel's comic book pages. As a human, Jennifer has no powers. But she can change into She-Hulk! She-Hulk is a powerful green superhero. She is strong, fast, and has amazing healing abilities. The angrier she is, the faster she heals herself!

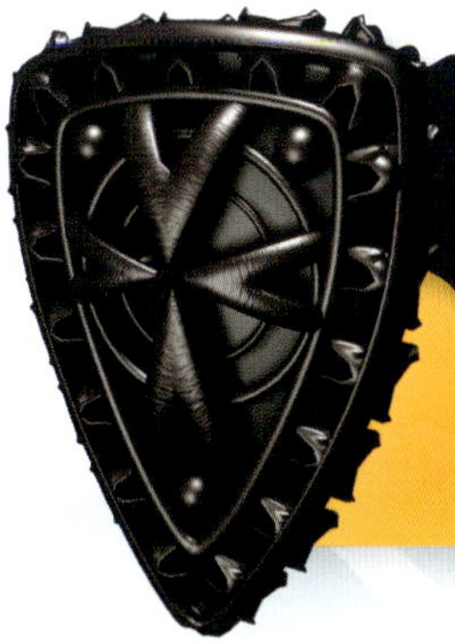

MADE OF STEEL

- Wolverine's skeleton is covered in adamantium. This fictional steel is nearly indestructible!

MEDIA MANIA!

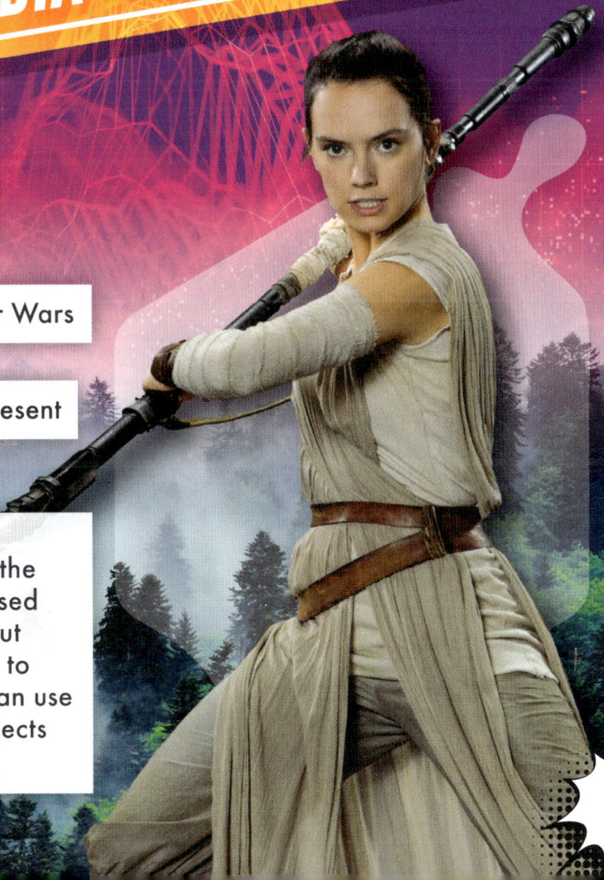

CHARACTER Rey

MOVIE SERIES Star Wars

YEARS 2015 to present

DESCRIPTION

Rey has the power of the Force. This power is used by the Jedi. Throughout the movies, Rey trains to become a Jedi. She can use the Force to move objects and heal people!

Cyborg appeared in DC Comics in the 1980s. He is part human and part robot. Cyborg is very strong and can control technology. He has a self-repair system. It repairs damaged parts of his robotic body. It can also heal parts of his human body. This repair system even makes upgrades!

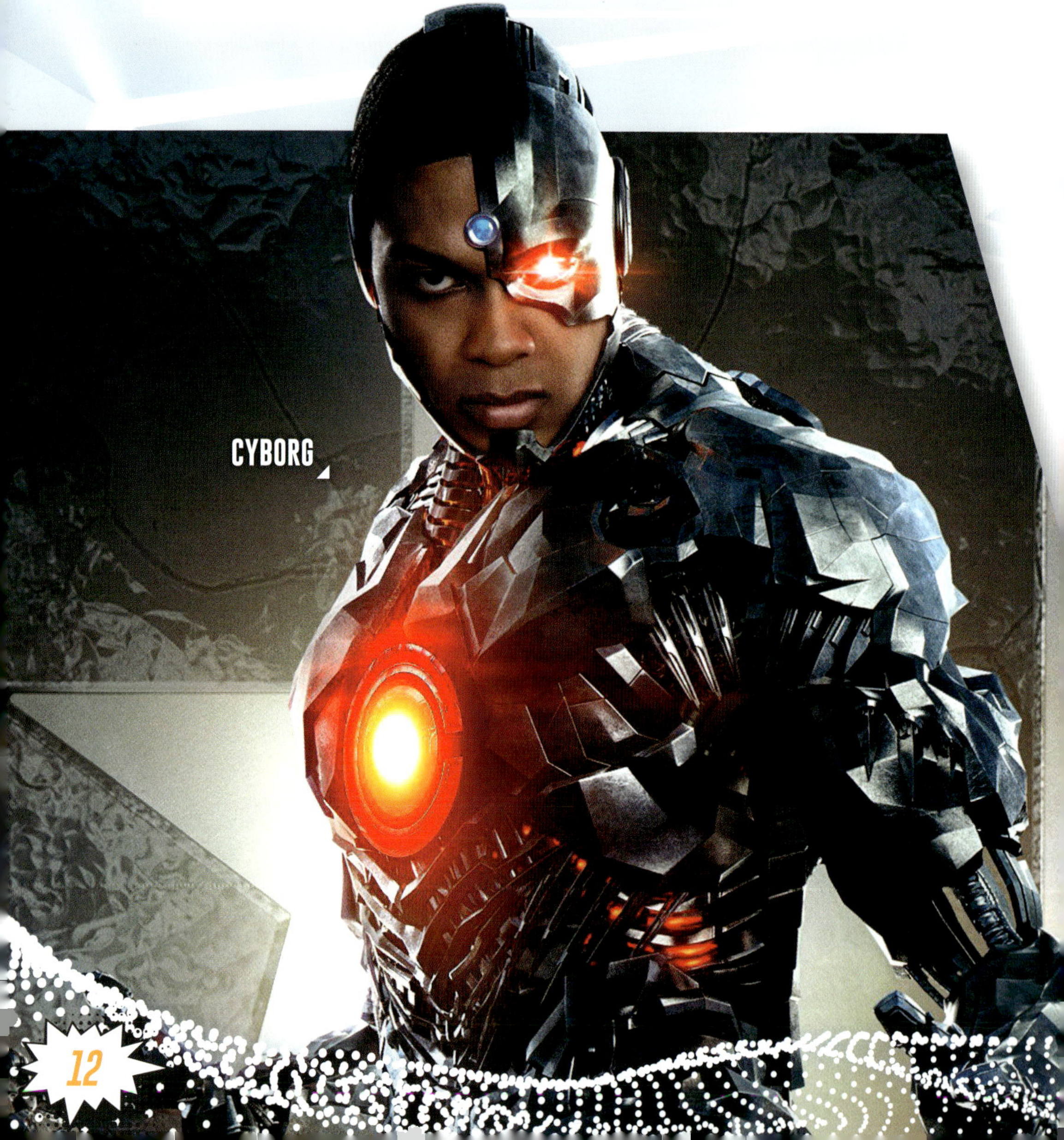

SUPERHERO PROFILE

SUPERHERO NAME Cyborg

REAL NAME Victor Stone

SUPERPOWERS

super healing, super strength, technology control, teleportation, genius-level intellect

BACKSTORY

When Victor was a teenager, he was in a deadly accident. His father used advanced technology to save Victor's life. As a result, Victor became part human, part robot. It gave him many powers including super strength, super healing, and technology control. He uses his powers to help others. He has been a member of the Teen Titans and the Justice League.

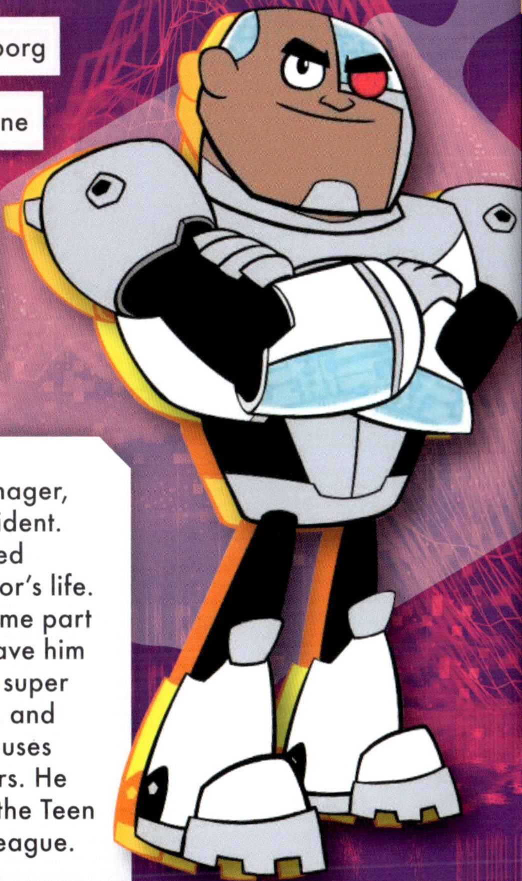

SELECT APPEARANCES

- *DC Comics Presents* issue number 26 (1980)
- *New Teen Titans* comics (1980 to 1984)
- *Teen Titans* TV series (2003 to 2006)
- *Teen Titans Go!* TV series (2013 to present)
- *Justice League* feature films (2017, 2021)

More recent heroes with super healing abilities include Marvel's Wiccan. He first appeared in comics in 2005. His mother is the Scarlet Witch. Like her, he can use magic to heal other people.

EVERYDAY HEALING

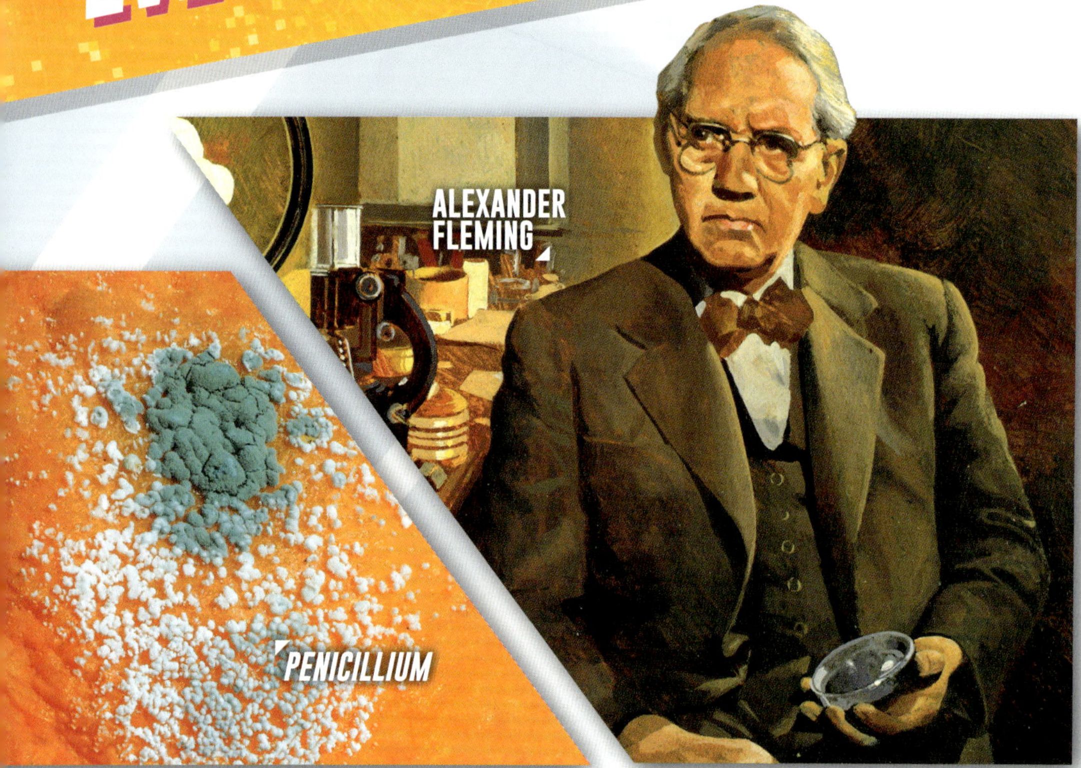

People have searched for many ways to heal themselves. In ancient times, people discovered that many plants have healing properties. Some relieved pain while others helped treat illnesses.

Nature has helped create a lot of modern medicines. In 1928, Alexander Fleming discovered a **mold** called *Penicillium*. The mold kept **bacteria** from being able to grow. Fleming used his discovery to create penicillin. It was the world's first **antibiotic**. Doctors use antibiotics today to help people fight **infections**.

THE POWER OF PLANTS

- People once used willow bark to relieve pain. It worked similar to modern pain relievers!

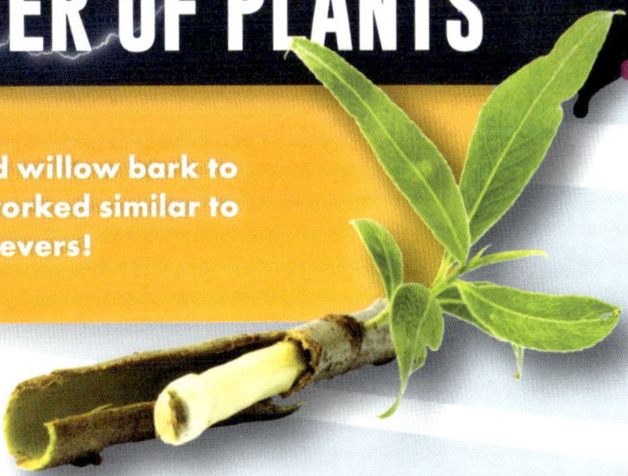

SUPER HEALING IN NATURE

SOME ANIMALS HAVE AMAZING HEALING ABILITIES!

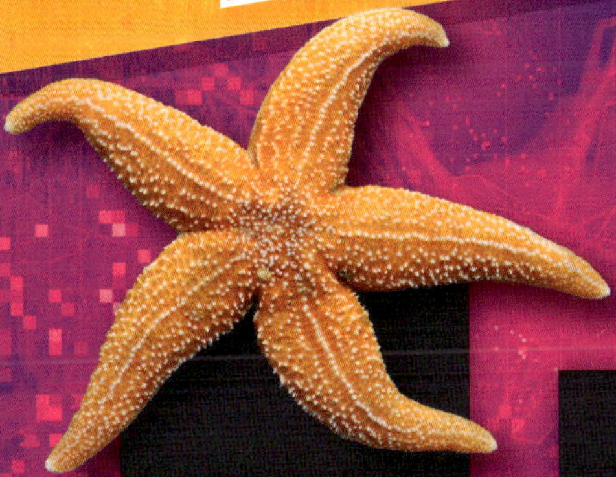

SEA STARS

SOME CAN REGROW AN ENTIRE BODY FROM A LOST LIMB

ZEBRAFISH

THEY CAN REPAIR DAMAGE TO THEIR OWN HEARTS

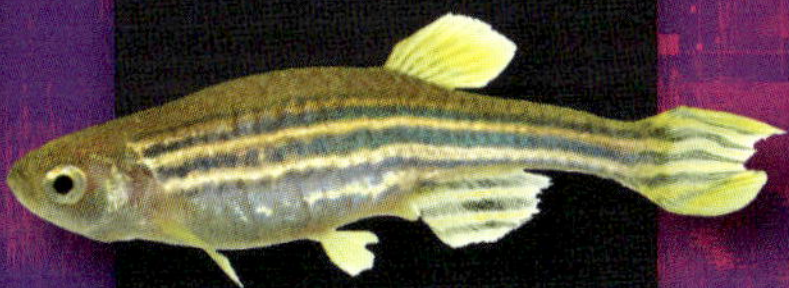

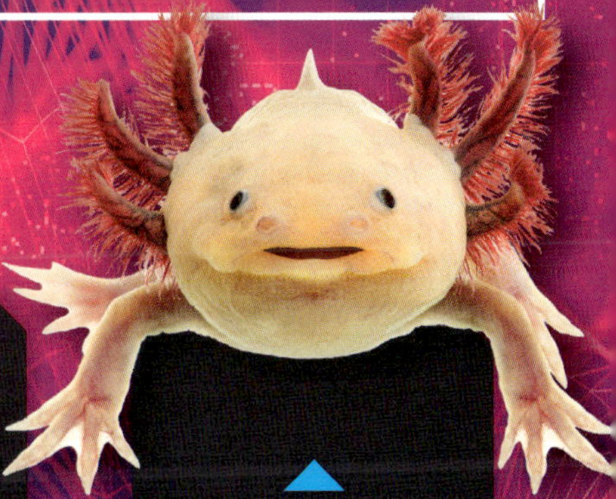

AXOLOTL

THEY CAN REGROW THEIR TAILS, LIMBS, AND EVEN PARTS OF THEIR BRAINS

Surgery is a medical practice that involves cutting into a person's body. Doctors perform surgery to treat diseases or serious cuts and wounds. Doctors can even replace body parts. In **transplant** surgery, they replace a damaged **organ**, such as a liver. They can replace joints such as hips or knees with metal or plastic parts.

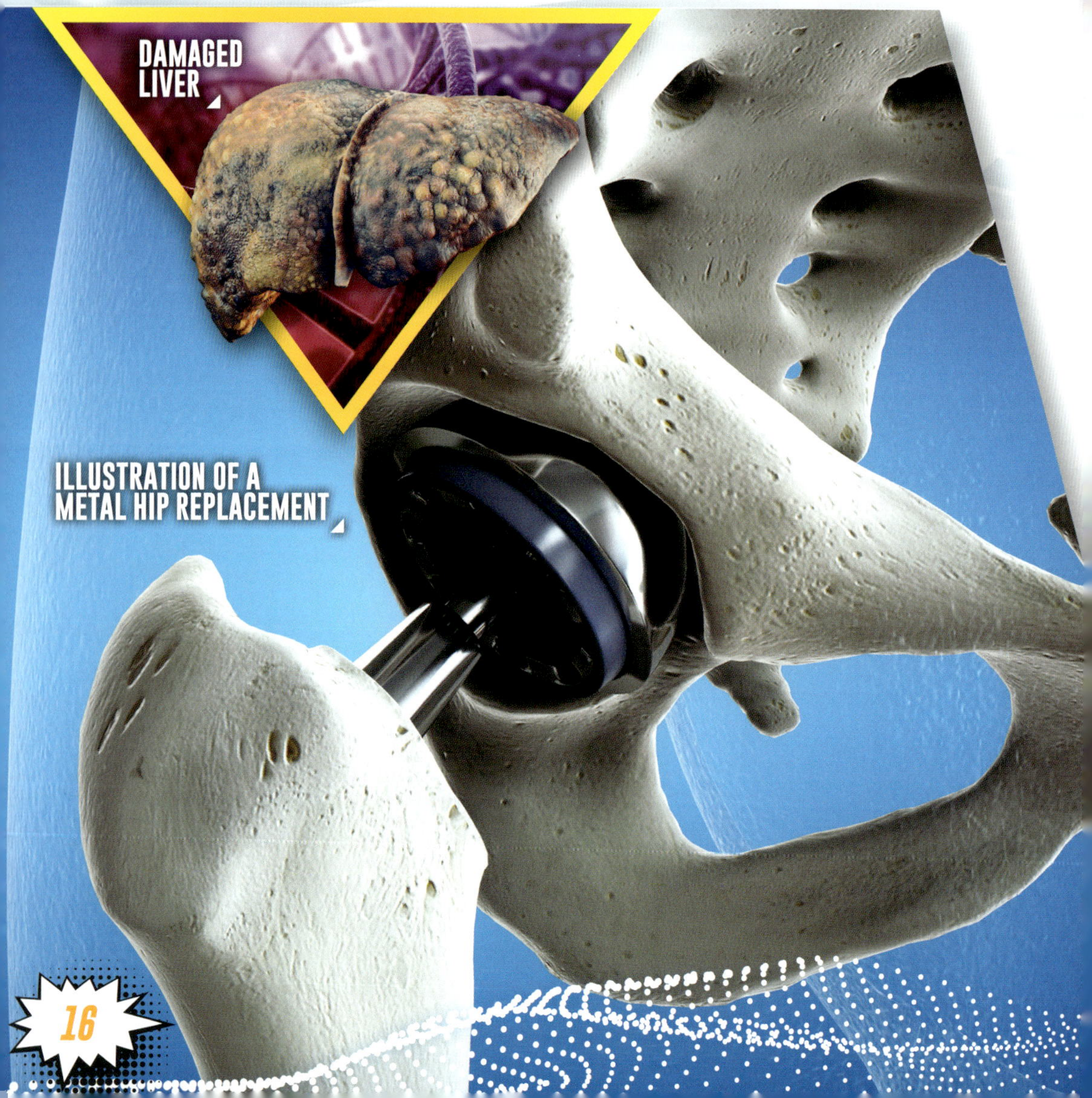

DAMAGED LIVER

ILLUSTRATION OF A METAL HIP REPLACEMENT

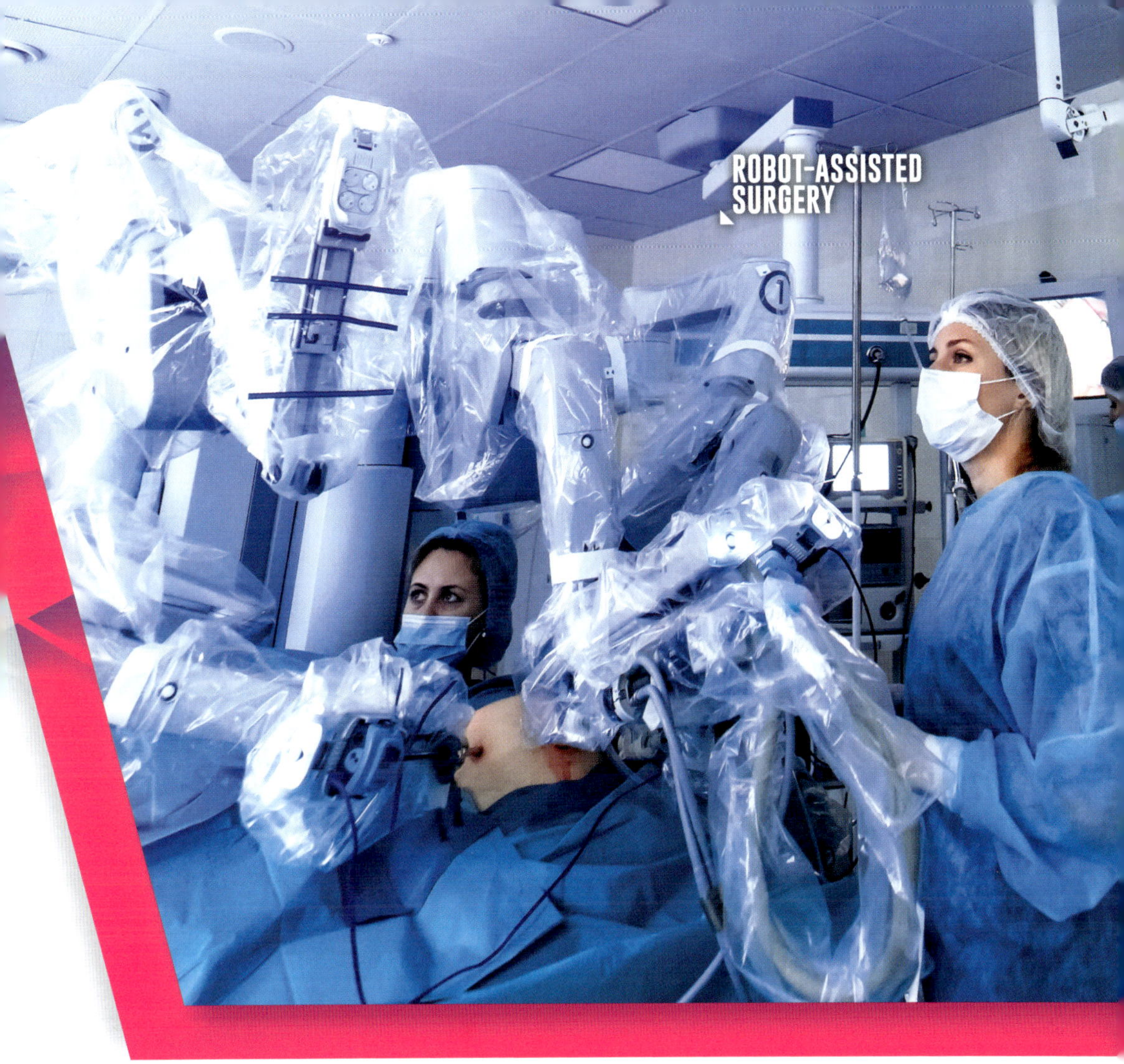

Today, many surgeries are performed with the aid of robots. A doctor controls robotic arms that hold surgical instruments. The robot arms can operate more accurately than a surgeon. Robot-assisted surgeries are often less painful. Patients also heal more quickly from them.

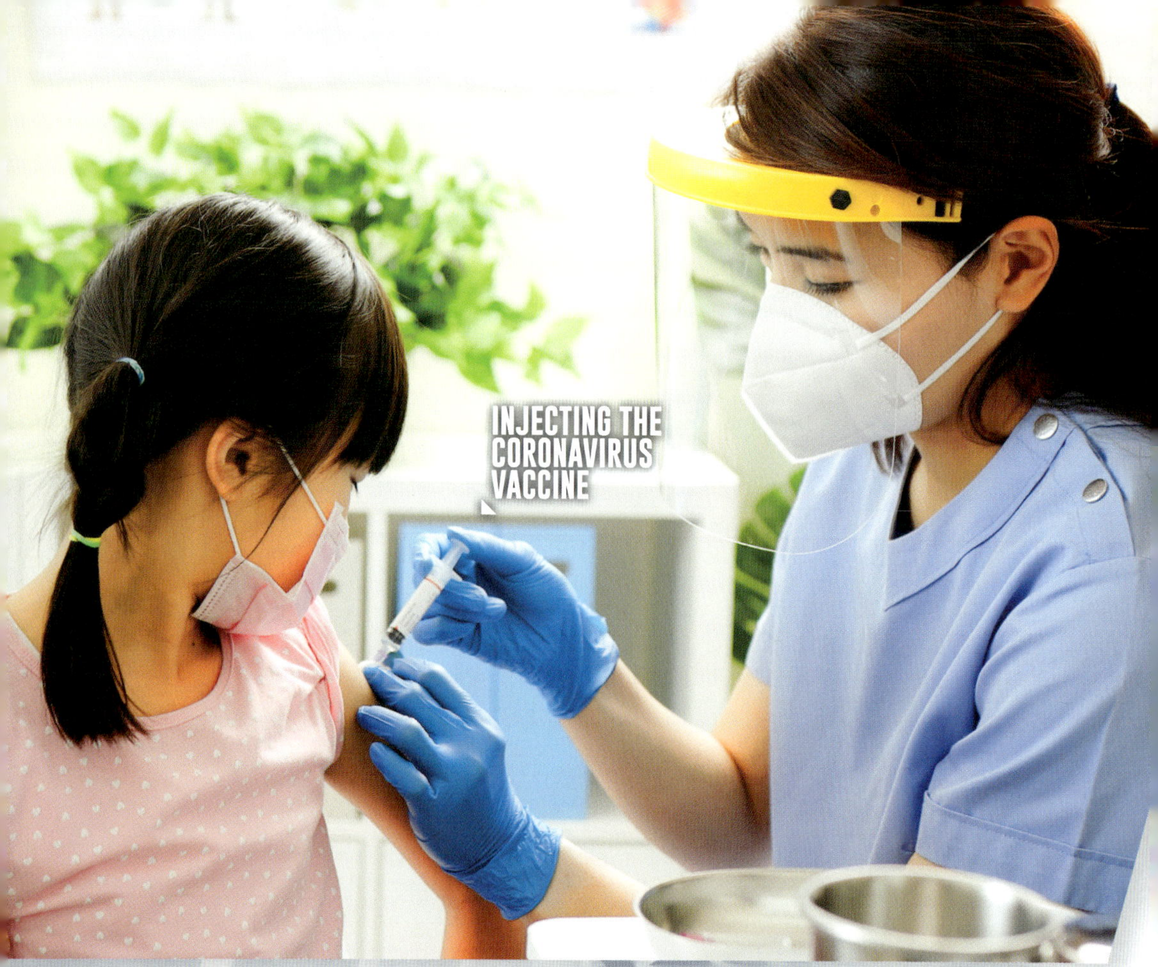

Doctors also give patients **vaccines** to strengthen the **immune system**. British physician Edward Jenner made the first vaccine in the 1790s to protect people from smallpox. Today, vaccines help prevent illnesses such as **coronavirus** and the flu.

Most vaccines contain dead or weakened germs of a disease. They are usually **injected** into a person with a needle. Vaccines make the immune system create **antibodies** to fight the germs in the vaccine. Then, the immune system remembers how to quickly fight off the disease in the future.

VACCINE ADVANCEMENTS

▸ Some of the coronavirus vaccines are mRNA vaccines. They do not contain any germs of the virus. Instead, the vaccines have substances that teach the immune system how to fight coronavirus.

THE SCIENCE BEHIND A VACCINE

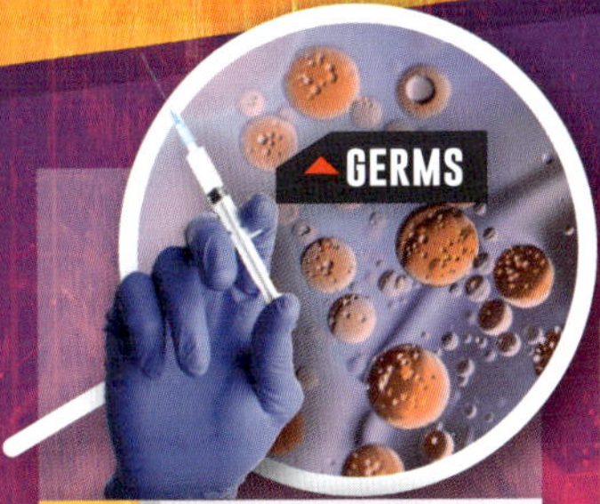

1 A vaccine contains dead or weakened germs

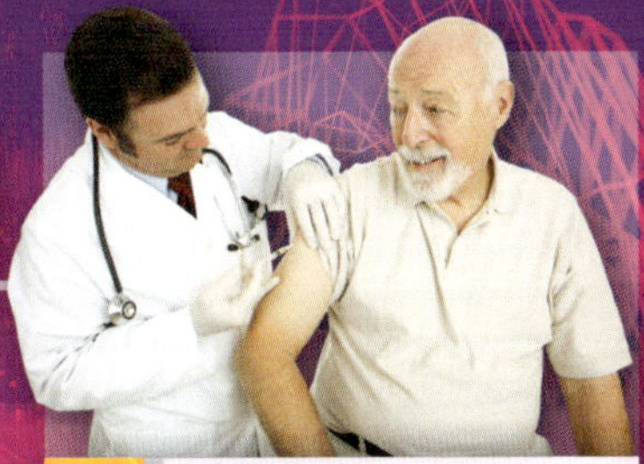

2 The vaccine is injected into a person's body with a needle

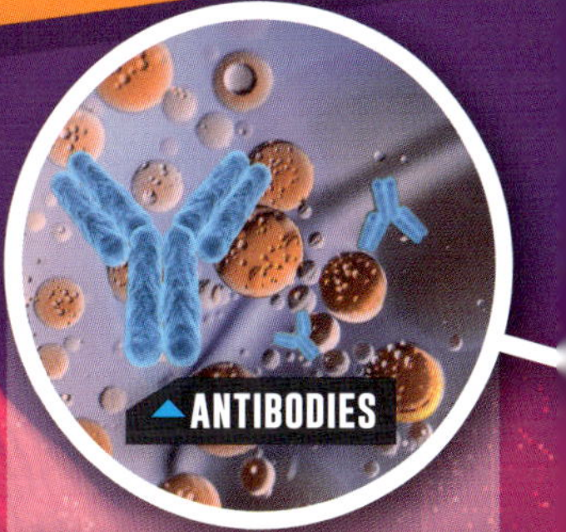

3 The immune system reacts to the germs and creates antibodies

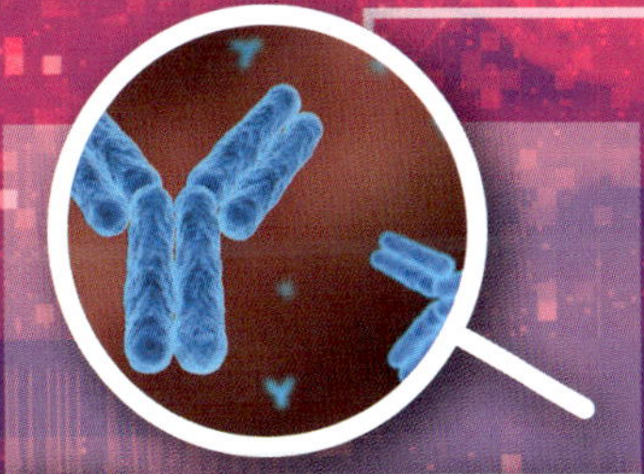

4 The antibodies attack and destroy the germs in the vaccine

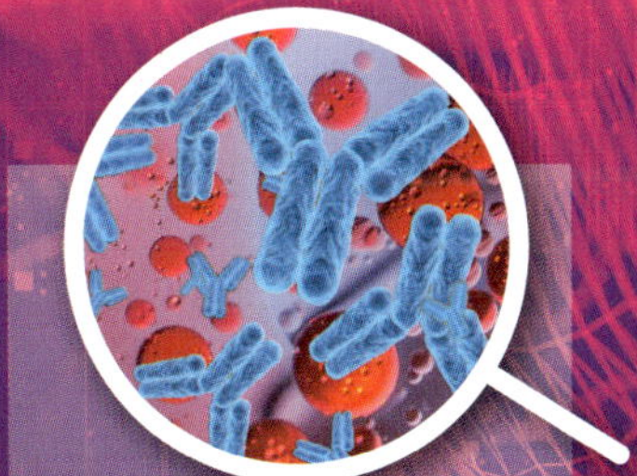

5 The immune system remembers how to fight off the germs for the future

IS SUPER HEALING POSSIBLE?

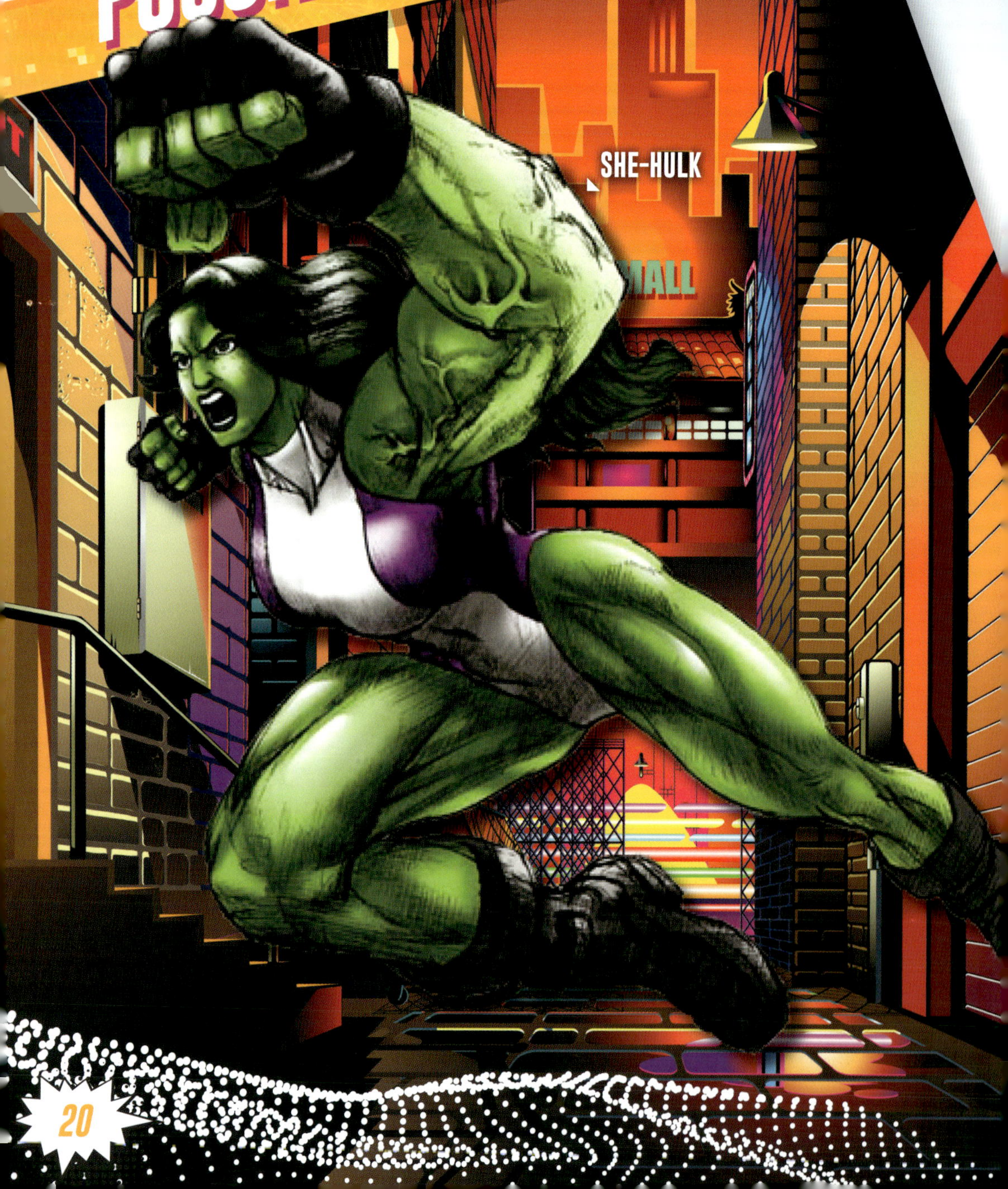

Superheroes are not as easily harmed as people. Some heroes are super tough like She-Hulk. They can withstand blows and blasts that would severely hurt a person. Other heroes can quickly heal themselves like the Flash or Wolverine.

Unlike many superheroes, people need time to heal. It can take a person months or even years to recover from a serious injury. Some people do not fully recover from injuries. People may also need **physical therapy**. This treatment helps a person recover from physical injuries.

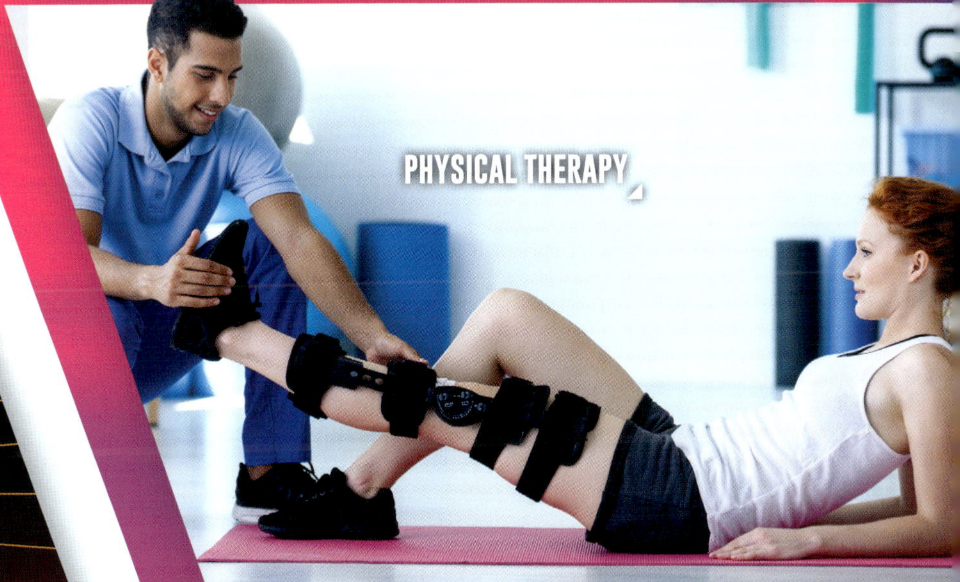

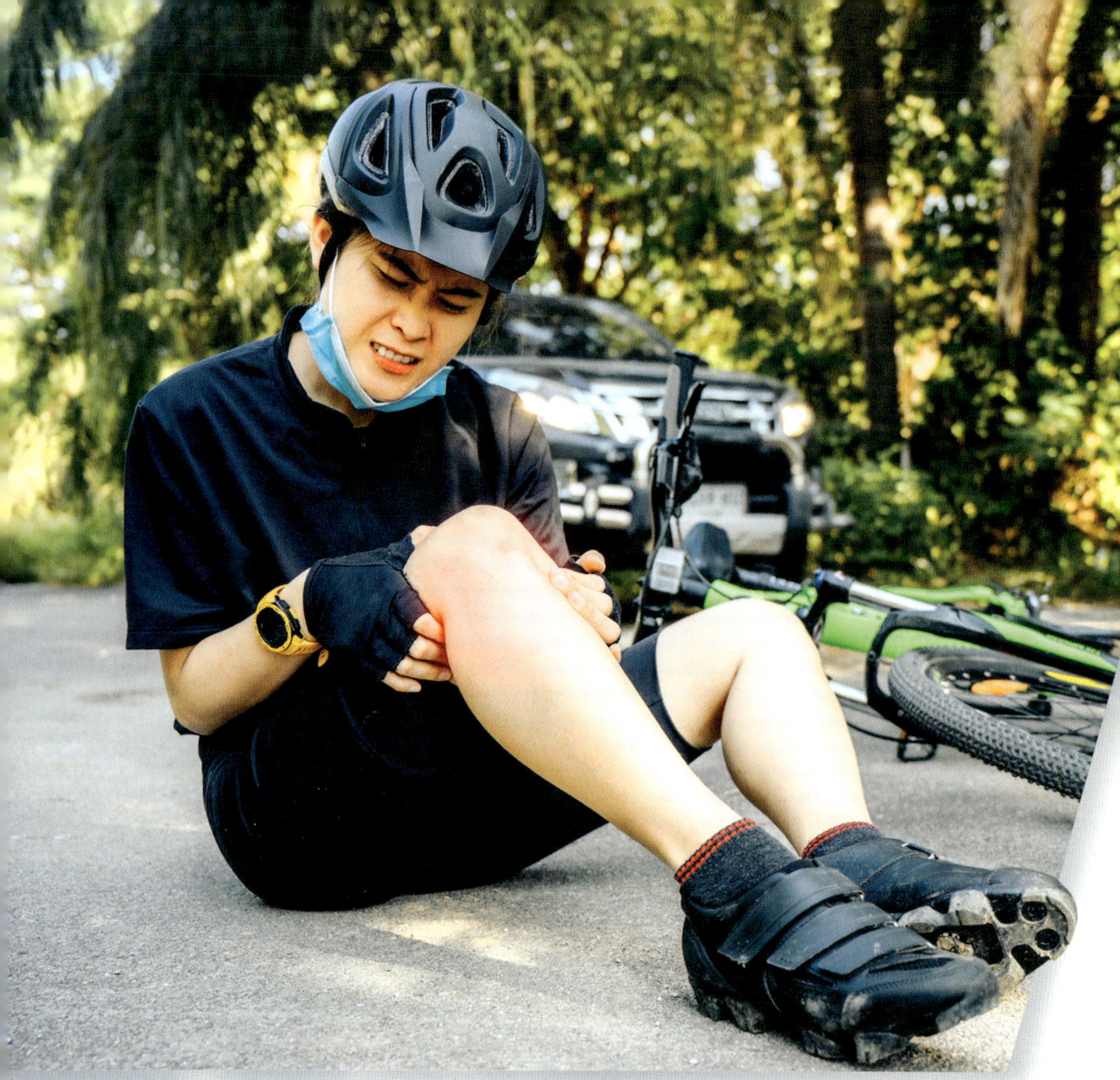

Even if people could quickly heal themselves, they would still feel pain. Serious injuries like burns or broken bones are very painful. Additionally, if injuries heal too quickly, they may heal incorrectly. For example, if a broken bone is not set correctly, it will heal wrong. It would cause more pain and other health issues.

If a person could heal from any illness or injury, they could be **immortal**. They would outlive friends and family. Over time, they might feel very lonely.

NEGATIVE EFFECTS OF SUPER HEALING

CAN HEAL FROM ANY INJURY

EFFECT: ▸ CAN STILL FEEL PAIN

HEAL QUICKLY

EFFECTS:
- MAY HEAL INCORRECTLY
- CAUSE MORE PAIN AND HEALTH ISSUES

IMMORTALITY

EFFECTS:
- OUTLIVE LOVED ONES
- LONELINESS

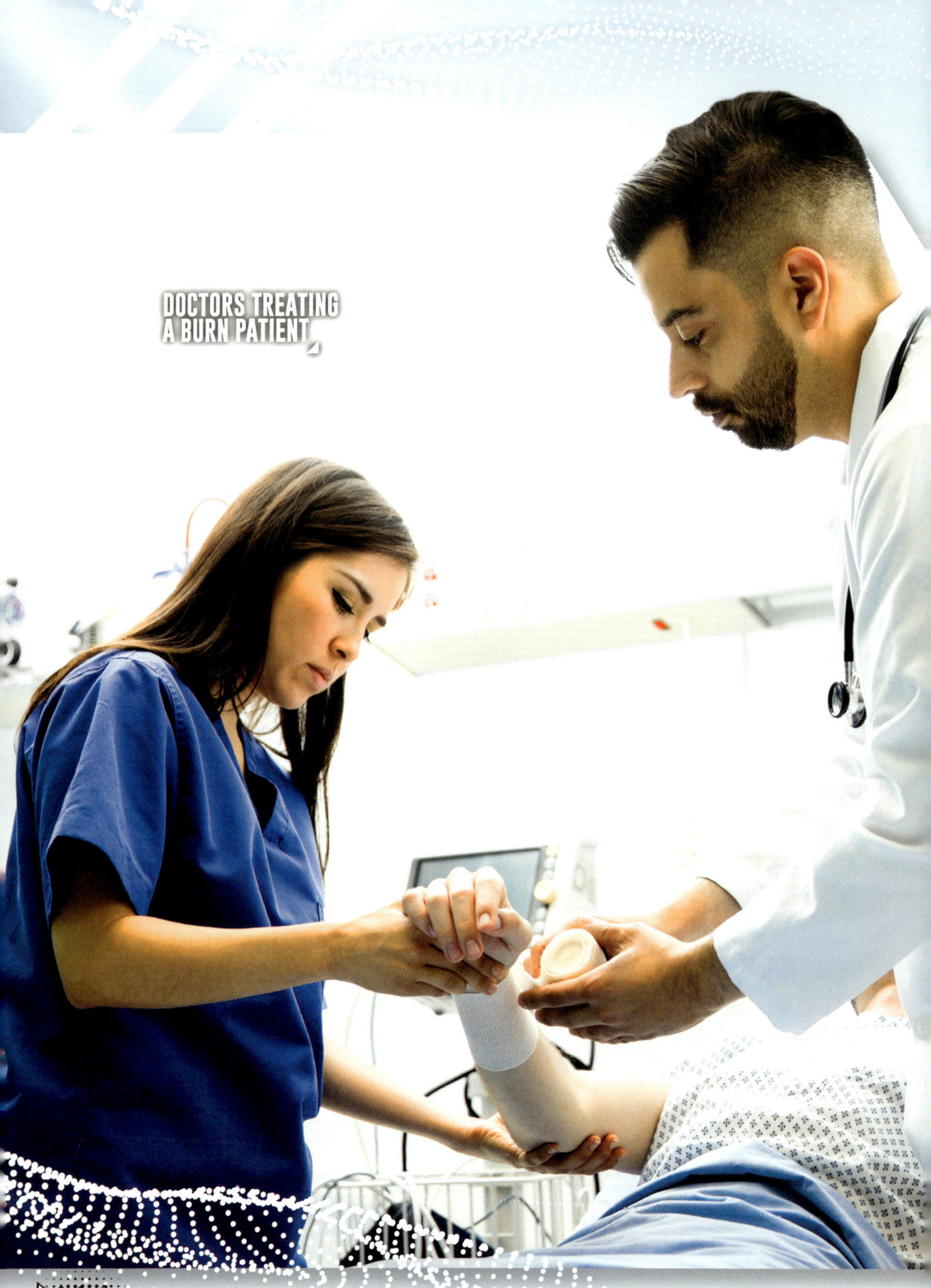

DOCTORS TREATING A BURN PATIENT

Doctors have found some amazing new ways to help people heal. To treat burns, some hospitals are using the RECELL System. This treatment was approved in 2018. It uses skin **cells** from a patient mixed with a special liquid. The mixture is sprayed on a patient's burns. This treatment helps patients heal faster. It also helps reduce scarring.

Special bandages can help speed up healing, too. NASA created bandages that use low levels of electricity. The electricity helps cells repair injuries at a faster rate.

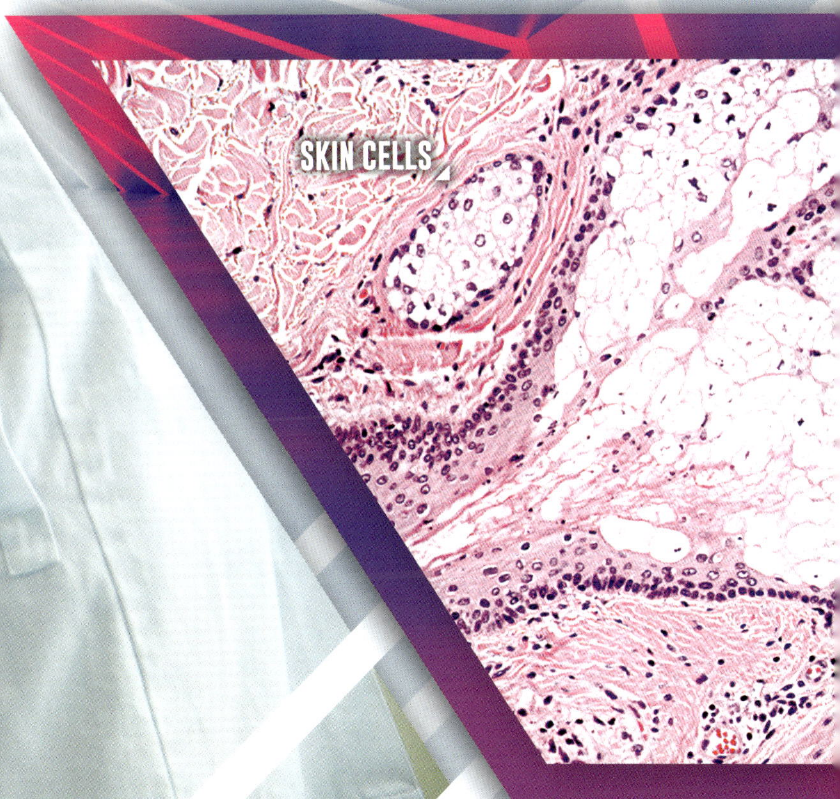

THE FUTURE OF HEALING

People will likely never have healing abilities like Wolverine or the Flash. They may not use magic like the Scarlet Witch to heal others, either. But scientists might create new medical practices with technology.

One way might be through **nanites**. Nanites are very small robots. They can be injected into a person's body. Nanites can be **programmed** to deliver medicine to specific parts of a person's body. They can also be made to repair injuries inside the body.

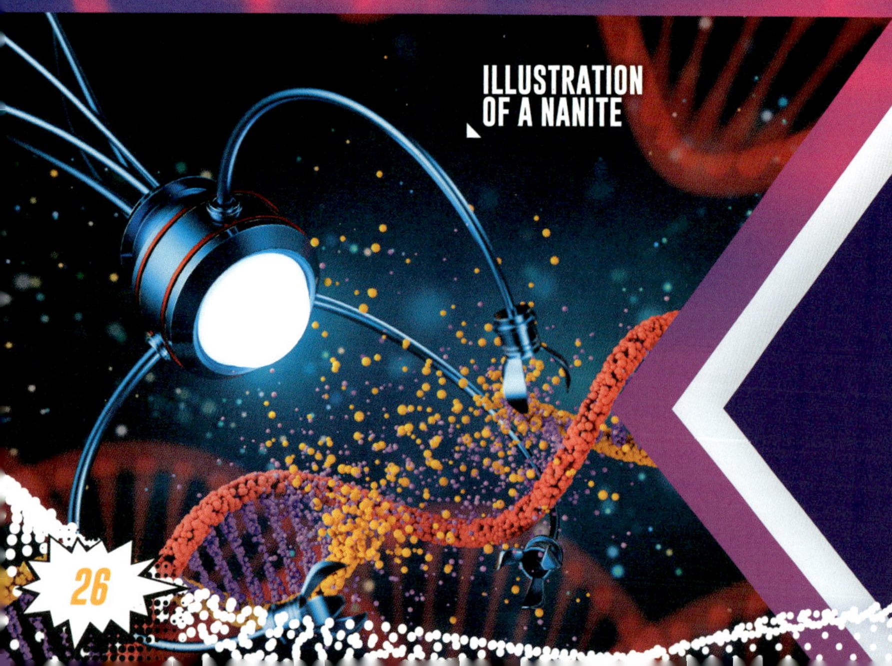

ILLUSTRATION OF A NANITE

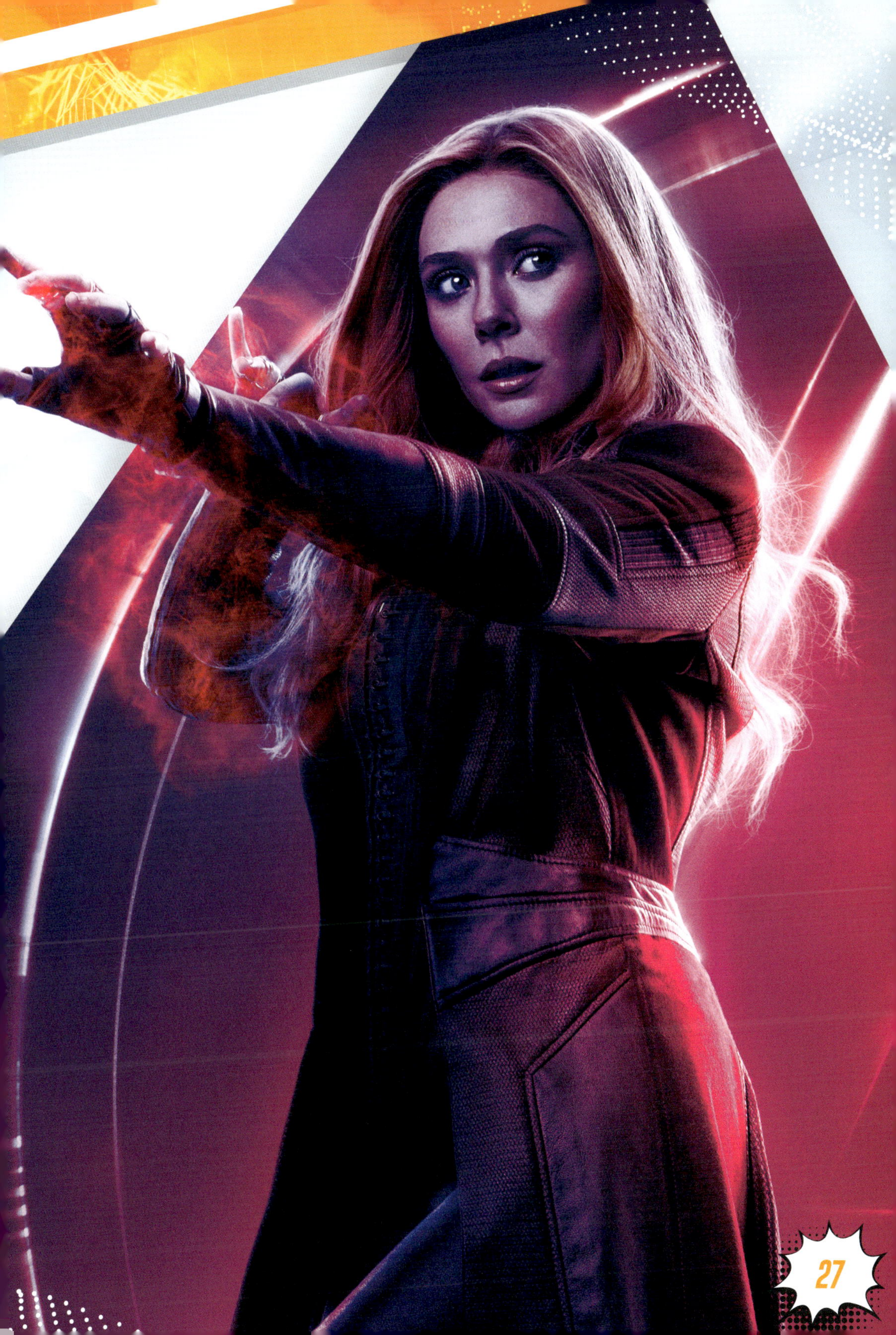

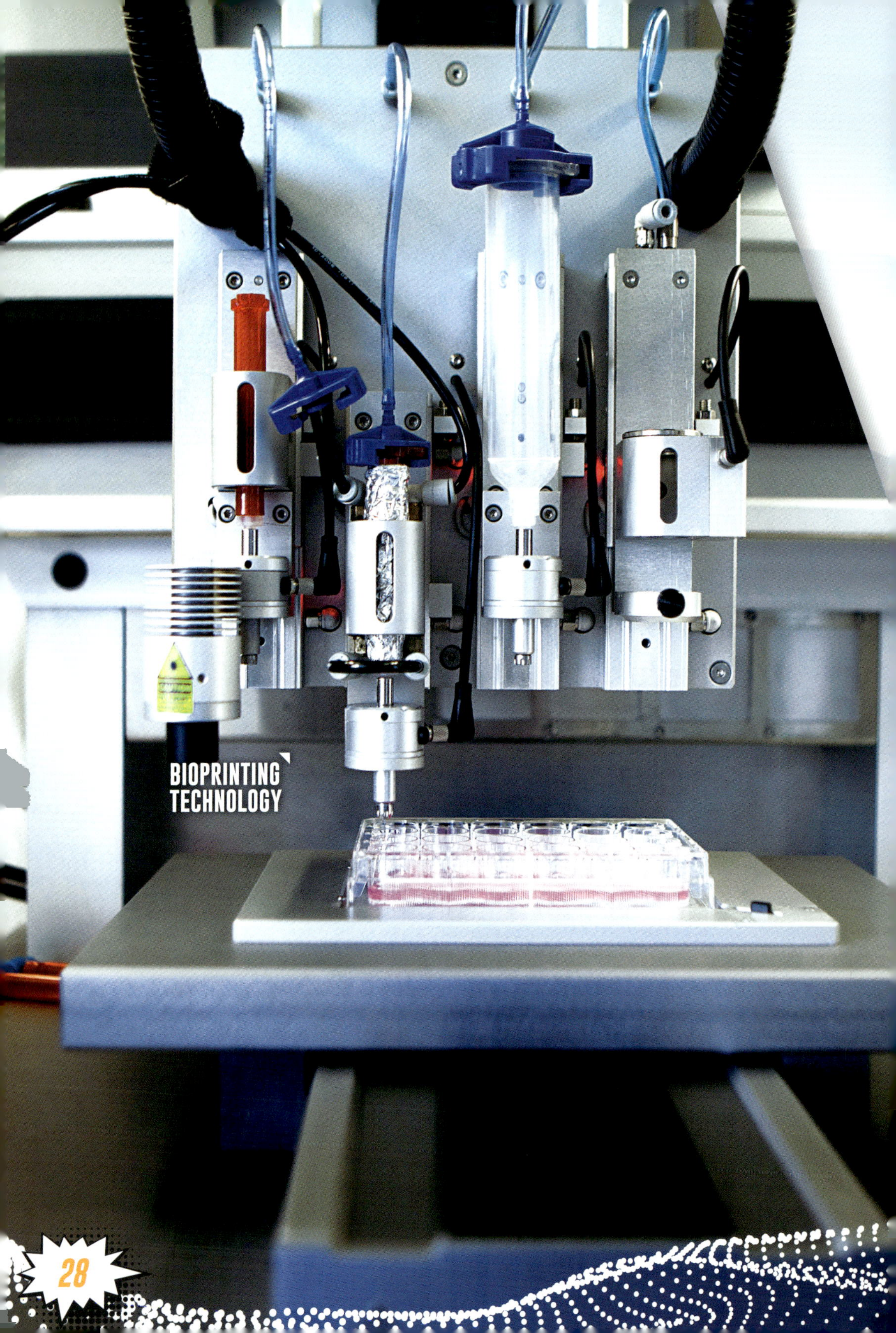

BIOPRINTING TECHNOLOGY

New technologies might help people who need organ transplants. Right now, patients can wait for years before receiving a **donated** organ. In the future, scientists might create new organs though **bioprinting**. This technology could create new organs or bones with a patient's cells. So far, scientists have created new skin cells and blood vessels.

People may never heal themselves like superheroes. But scientists are finding new ways to help people heal. One day, new technologies could fully heal people from severe injuries and deadly diseases!

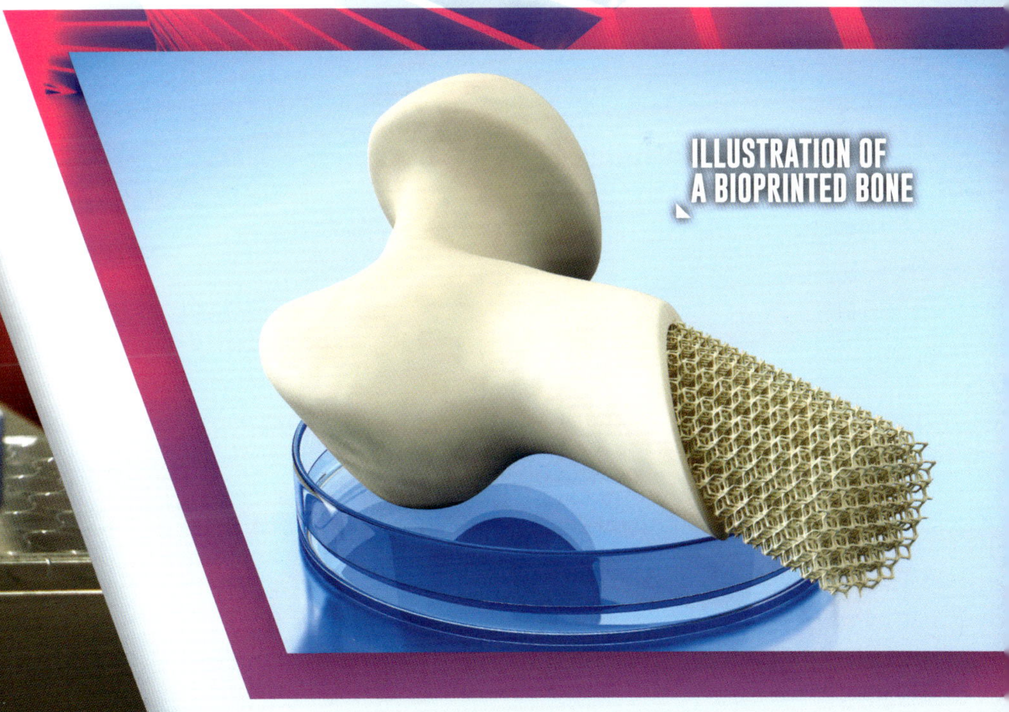
ILLUSTRATION OF A BIOPRINTED BONE

GLOSSARY

ability–the power to do something

antibiotic–a medicine that prevents small, harmful organisms from growing

antibodies–parts of a person's immune system that fight against diseases

bacteria–small living things that sometimes can cause illnesses in people

bioprinting–the use of 3D printing technology to create organs and tissues using living cells and nonliving materials

cells–the smallest units of living things

coronavirus–a deadly illness that causes coughing, loss of smell and taste, and difficulty breathing

donated–given to someone from someone else

immortal–unable to die

immune system–a body system that fights infections and diseases in the human body

infections–diseases caused by germs

injected–put into the body through a needle

mold–an often fuzzy surface growth of fungus on a damp material

nanites–very tiny robots

organ–a body part that has a certain function such as the heart, liver, or lungs

physical therapy–the treatment of a disease or an injury of the muscles or joints that includes massages and exercises

programmed–given a set of instructions

sorcerer–a person who uses magic

transplant–related to the practice of removing one thing and replacing it with something else; transplant surgeries involve a person receiving an organ from another person.

vaccines–substances that are usually injected into a person or animal to protect against certain diseases

TO LEARN MORE

AT THE LIBRARY

Polinsky, Paige V. *Super Strength*. Minneapolis, Minn.: Bellwether Media, 2021.

Polinsky, Paige V. *Vaccines: A Graphic History*. Minneapolis, Minn.: Graphic Universe, 2022.

Rowell, Ronan. *Robots in Medicine*. New York, N.Y.: Cavendish Square Publishing, 2022.

ON THE WEB

FACTSURFER

Factsurfer.com gives you a safe, fun way to find more information.

1. Go to www.factsurfer.com.

2. Enter "super healing" into the search box and click .

3. Select your book cover to see a list of related content.

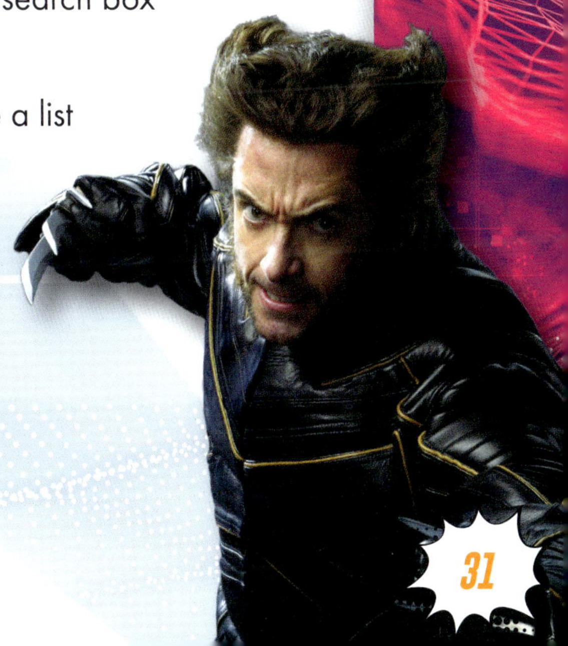

INDEX

The images in this book are reproduced through the courtesy of: ZUMA Press, Inc./ Alamy, front cover (Wolverine); Entertainment Pictures/ Alamy, pp. 3, 4-5 (Scarlet Witch), 31 (Wolverine); AF Archive/ Alamy, pp. 5 (Quicksilver), 6-7 (Ultron), 12-13 (Cyborg); Walt Disney Studios Motion Pictures/ Everett Collection, p. 6 (Hawkeye); Album/ Alamy, pp. 8-9, 14 (Alexander Fleming); Puwadol Jaturawutthichai, p. 9 (broken bone); cineclassico/ Alamy, pp. 10-11 (Wolverine); Mariusz Lubkowski, p. 11 (adamantium); Photo 12/ Alamy, p. 11 (Rey); MikeCloudStock, p. 11 (forest); AA Film Archive/ Alamy, p. 13 (Cyborg comic); Kateryna Kon, p. 14 (*penicillium*); shansh23, p. 15 (willow bark); Christian Musat, p. 15 (sea stars); David Dohnal, p. 15 (zebrafish); Eric Isselee, p. 15 (axoltol); eranicle, p. 16 (damaged liver); SciePro, pp. 16-17 (hip replacement); aslysun, p. 18 (injecting coronavirus vaccine); Prostock-studio, p. 19 (step 1 needle); Oscar Sweep, p. 19 (step 1, 3, 5 germs); Lisa F. Young, p. 19 (step 2); Jason Busa, p. 19 (step 3, 4, 5 antibodies); Kiriti_yuda, pp. 20-21 (She-Hulk); creativica, pp. 20-21 (background); Photography.eu, p. 21 (physical therapy); Boyloso, pp. 22-23; antoniodiaz, pp. 24-25 (burn patient); Cultura RM/ Alamy, p. 25 (skin cells); K_E_N, p. 26 (nanite); TCD/Prod.DB/ Alamy, pp. 26-27 (Scarlet Witch); BSIP SA/ Alamy, p. 28 (bioprinting technology); Iaremenko Sergii, p. 29 (bioprinted bone).